FASTING 101

Your Complete Guide to Intermittent Fasting, Alternative Day Fasting, the benefits and more.

ELLIE PERICO

Thank you for purchasing my book & supporting my passion for helping others learn about nutrition and overall health! I hope you find it to be informative and helpful. If you purchased the hard copy and do not have access to the links, I can send them to you via email (ellieperico@aol.com), via direct message on Instagram (@fitcopmom) or you can find them on my You Tube channel by searching my name or handle @fitcopmom.

If you have any other questions, I'm always available to help answer them and/or help guide you in your health and fitness journey! Answering questions is free & I'm happy to do so but I also provide one on one and group coaching. If you're interested, contact me via email or Instagram.

If you're interested in learning about macros, how to calculate them for your goals, track them easily in an app & use them to help guide you in your fitness journey while fasting, see my Macros 101 book. It is also available as an ebook and a hard copy, has received great reviews and has helped many reach their goals. Fasting and tracking calories & macros go hand in hand. Just because you are fasting doesn't mean you can eat as much and anything you want so you'll find it helpful if you're serious about changing your health for the better! Thanks again! I appreciate your support more than you know!

Ellie Perico

Contents

WHAT IS FASTING

Fasting is when you willfully refrain from eating for a certain amount of time. This can be hours or days. True fasting means you do not eat or drink anything other than water, black coffee or plain unflavored tea. If you are fasting under doctor's orders for a blood test or other medical procedure he/she may suggest consuming nothing other than water. But for weightloss and/or health purposes, water, unflavored club soda, black coffee and plain, unflavored tea (green is recommended) is allowed. Stevia is allowed in very amounts. Click https://youtu.be/CGWl2lbUDS4 to watch a short video I made on an introduction to fasting, benefits, allowed beverages and more before continuing with the book.

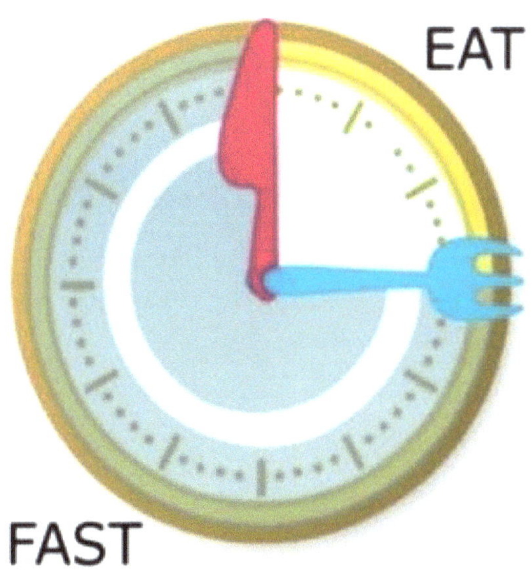

FASTING HEALTH BENEFITS

Fasting is a practice that has been associated with many health benefits outside of possible weight loss if done correctly.

One of the most common benefits of fasting is the stimulation of autophagy. It will be discussed further in the book because it is one of the main reasons I fast & most important benefits in my opinion.. Below that are the many other benefits that come with fasting as well. .

Regeneration of Cells through Autophagy

Autophagy is a process in which old parts of cells are degraded and recycled. It plays a key role in preventing diseases, including cancer, neurodegeneration, heart disease, and infections.

Animal studies have shown that long- and short-term fasting increase autophagy and are linked to delayed aging, a reduced risk of tumors & increased lifespan[1].

This has been supported by human studies showing that alternate day fasting reduces oxidative damage and promotes changes that may be linked to longevity.

---

1   https://www.ncbi.nlm.nih.gov/pmc/articles/PMC3919445/

Boost Heart Health by Improving Blood Pressure, Triglyceride and Cholesterol Levels

Heart disease is considered the leading cause of death in the United States and around the world. Some research has found that incorporating intermittent or alternate day fasting into your routine may be beneficial when it comes to improving heart health.

One study revealed that eight weeks of alternate-day fasting reduced levels of "bad" LDL cholesterol 25% and triglycerides by 32% [2].

A study in 4,629 people associated fasting with a lower risk of coronary artery disease, as well as a significantly lower risk of diabetes, which is a major risk factor for heart disease[3].

Helps Reduce Inflammation

Inflammation has been linked to serious health conditions such as heart disease, cancer and rheumatoid arthritis. Studies have shown that by incorporating fasting, one can significantly decrease inflammation in the body, leading to improved treatment of chronic inflammatory diseases such as multiple sclerosis.

One study among 50 healthy adults showed that intermittent fasting for one month significantly decreased levels of inflammatory markers[4].

---

2   https://pubmed.ncbi.nlm.nih.gov/20300080/

3   https://www.ncbi.nlm.nih.gov/pmc/articles/PMC2572991/

4   https://pubmed.ncbi.nlm.nih.gov/23244540/

Improved Brain Function and Aids in Prevention of Neurodegenerative Disorders

Like many other areas of research, studies are mostly limited to animals but several have found that fasting seems to have a positive effect on brain function.

A study in mice showed that intermittent fasting improved both brain function and structure (Source).

Because fasting also helps relieve inflammation, it could also aid in preventing neurodegenerative disorders such as Alzheimer's disease and Parkinson's

Increases Growth Hormone Secretion

Human growth hormone (HGH) is a type of protein hormone that is vital to many aspects of your health. This key hormone is involved in growth, metabolism, weight loss and muscle strength.

Several studies have found that fasting could naturally increase human growth hormone levels. One study revealed that fasting for 24 hours significantly increased levels of HGH[5].

Another small study among men found that fasting for just 48 hours led to an increase of human growth hormone production at 5 times the normal rate[6].

---

5   https://pubmed.ncbi.nlm.nih.gov/22386777/

6   https://pubmed.ncbi.nlm.nih.gov/1548337/

Aids in Boosting Metabolism

Weight loss, reducing calorie intake and boosting metabolism are typically the reasons most people decide to take up fasting. It makes sense to think that abstaining from eating or drinking for a certain amount of time each day or certain days of each week would decrease your overall calorie intake, leading to increased weight loss over time

Some research has also found that short-term fasting may boost metabolism by increasing levels of the neurotransmitter norepinephrine, which could enhance weight loss[7].

In fact, one review showed that whole-day fasting could reduce body weight by up to 9% and significantly decrease body fat over 12–24 weeks[8].

There has also been some debate about fasting when it comes to fat and muscle loss. But research shows that fasting may increase metabolism while helping reduce body weight and fat and simultaneously helping preserve muscle tissue[9].

Aids in Cancer Prevention and Increased Effectiveness of Chemotherapy

Although most cancer research when it comes to fasting has been limited to to animals and cells, outcomes have been

---

7   https://pubmed.ncbi.nlm.nih.gov/10837292/

8   https://pubmed.ncbi.nlm.nih.gov/26374764/

9   https://pubmed.ncbi.nlm.nih.gov/21410865/

promising that fasting may aid in cancer prevention and increased effectiveness of chemotherapy in humans. One study conducted with rats found that alternate-day fasting helped block the formation of tumors[10].

A cell study showed that exposing cancer cells to cycles of fasting was as effective as chemotherapy in delaying tumor growth and increased the effectiveness of chemotherapy drugs on cancer formation[11].

Reduces Insulin Resistance & Helps Control Blood Sugar

Fasting has been shown to improve blood sugar levels and insulin resistance which is especially useful for those at risk of diabetes.

In a study of 10 individuals diagnosed with type 2 diabetes, those that incorporated short-term intermittent fasting into their lifestyle had significantly decreased blood sugar levels[12].

Another study found that both intermittent fasting and alternate-day fasting were equally effective at limiting calorie intake as they were at reducing insulin resistance[13].

What is important to note is that intermittent fasting and alternate day fasting affect men and women differently.

---

10   https://pubmed.ncbi.nlm.nih.gov/11835290/

11   https://www.ncbi.nlm.nih.gov/pmc/articles/PMC3608686/

12   https://www.ncbi.nlm.nih.gov/pmc/articles/PMC5394735/

13   https://pubmed.ncbi.nlm.nih.gov/24993615/

What works for some may not work for others. It's impor-tant to try both types and see if one and/or both work for you, your lifestyle, your goals and your current health situa-tion.

Help Delay Aging and Extend Longevity

Current research when it comes to aging has been limited to animal studies, however, results have shown to be promising in increased longevity and slowing the aging process.

In a study involving rats, fasting every other day delayed the rate of aging and helped them live 83% longer than rats that didn't fast[14].

---

14   https://pubmed.ncbi.nlm.nih.gov/7117847/

AUTOPHAGY

For most of my 46 years, I never considered fasting. I always thought starving the body for that long slowed down your metabolism & was an "unhealthy" thing to do, mostly because that's what "modern medicine" & mainstream media suggest. But after researching it, I started intermittent fasting, then completed my first 48 hr fast and have felt a considerable difference in my body, energy, mood, hunger, cravings & physical appearance ever since.

The benefits of fasting, as explained in the section above, are incredible. But Autophagy is, by far, in my opinion, the most valuable, both intermittently and with extended fasts.

While there are no exact rules/recommendations yet, researchers agree that extended fasting for autophagy, going for 24-72 hours without food ,is something that healthy people SHOULD do 2 or 3 times a year, ideally after getting your blood levels checked, to make sure they're not deficient in anything prior to starting

The idea behind autophagy is that, in the absence of external sources of food, the body begins to eat itself (auto: self, phage: eat), destroying & recycling its own damaged cells & proteins, so that new, healthy versions can be built. Autophagy is believed to be essential for helping protect against diseases like cancer & dementia, reduce inflammation, improve daily bodily function, prevent or delay neurodegenerative diseases, increase longevity & reverse signs of aging.

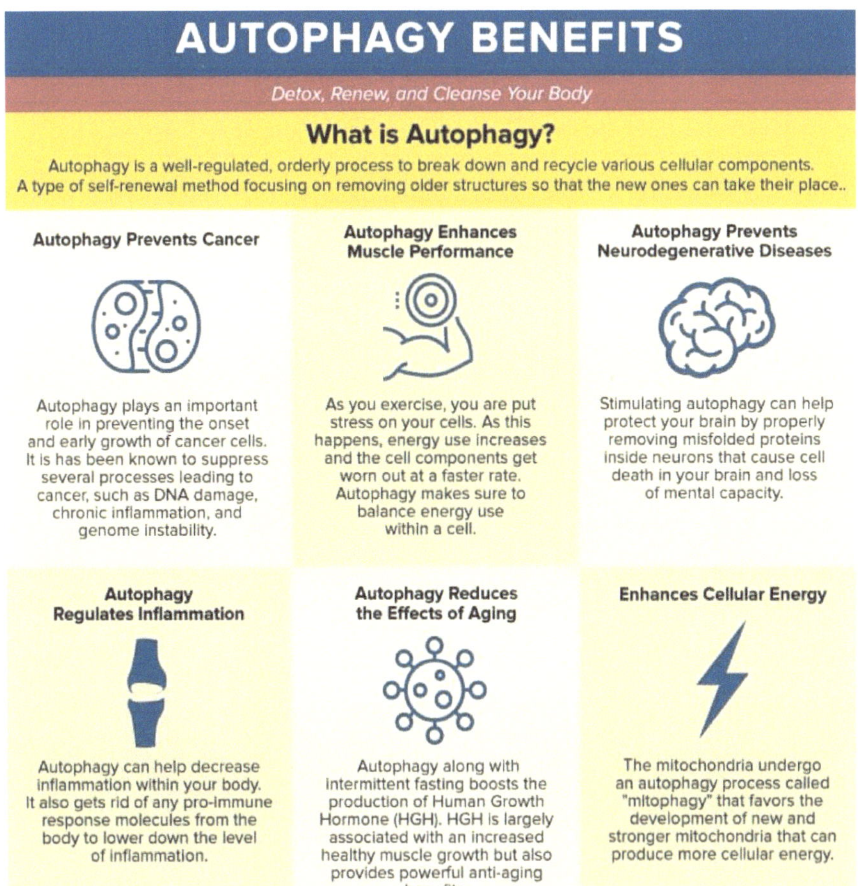

Animal studies have consistently shown that long- and short-term fasting that induces autophagy are linked to delayed aging, a reduced risk of tumors, an increase the lifespan and may help keep you healthy and live longer.

This has been supported by human studies showing that ADF (alternate day fasting) diets reduce oxidative damage and promote changes that may be linked to longevity[15].

---

15 https://pubmed.ncbi.nlm.nih.gov/15640462/

TYPES OF FASTING

There are several different types of fasting and, for the sake of making it easier for most to understand, I will be breaking it down into 3 categories. Intermittent Fasting, Alternate Day Fasting and Extended Fasting.

Intermittent Fasting

Intermittent fasting has gained popularity over the last few years and it is commonly practiced daily by many. If you want to begin fasting, this is the best method to ease into it with.

Intermittent fasting is when you do not eat anything or drink anything other than water, black coffee or green tea for a certain number of hours each day.

The most common method is the 16:8. This means your eating window is 8 hours each day and you do not eat for the remaining 16 hours of the day. It seems like a long time to go without eating but your eating window SHOULD include 8 hours of sleep and ideally 4 hours before going to bed and 4 hours once you wake up. This breaks up the non-eating window to make it more doable for most, however, how you break up the 16 hours is up to you, your lifestyle and your work schedule. You will have to take into account when you exercise, how late you stay up, how early you wake up and when you are most likely to feel hunger.

INTERMITTENT FASTING
MADE SIMPLE 👌

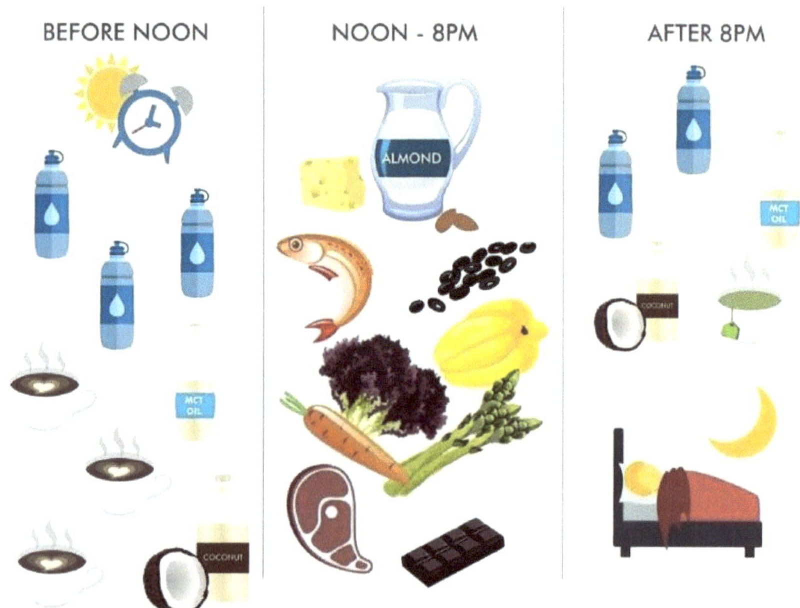

FASTING/EATING WINDOWS CAN VARY BUT THIS IS THE MOST COMMON 16:8 FOR A REGULAR 9-5 SCHEDULE

For example, my eating window is usually 1pm (1300 hrs) to 9pm (2100 hrs) but It changes depending on my schedule and/or if I am on the road or traveling. With the 1pm to 9pm schedule, it means after 9 pm I usually stop eating and I don't eat again until after 1pm the following day. I do this MOST days of the week. I do, at times, break this, usually weekends when I'm out late. I might shift it to 2pm to 10pm,

4pm to midnight or sometimes just shorten my fasting window to 14 hours and fast 14:8 instead. I chose the 1-9pm window primarily because I'm usually not hungry in the morning and I prefer to exercise on an empty stomach. I also do not get up very early and I stay up late.

If you go to bed very early, rise earlier and tend to prefer eating breakfast and avoiding food later in the evening, your window may be 9am to 5pm, 10am to 6pm, etc.

If you are just starting with intermittent fasting, you can start with a shorter fasting window and work your way up to 16:8. Many begin at 12:12, eat for 12 and fast for 12. Then graduate to 14:10 and then 16.8. An option more advanced after 16:8 is 20:4. The eating window is only 4 hours and the fasting window is 20 hours.

As far as meals are concerned, it is up to you if you want to have 3 solid meals as usual or smaller meals throughout your eating window with snacks mixed in. The numbers of meals and/or snacks does not matter, just like it doesn't matter even when you aren't fasting. What matters is that you are only eating in your eating window and that you stay in your daily caloric requirement and macro window. For more information on that, see my[16].

OMAD or One Meal A Day is a form of intermittent fasting where you fast for 23 hours and eat for the same 1-hour window each day. It's recommended you consume your one

---

16   https://amzn.to/3o0D4Q0

meal each day after your most active part of the day. This is a very restrictive type of fasting and typically done for weight loss. It is difficult to adhere to and not much more beneficial health wise than alternate day fasting or 20:4, 23:1 intermittent fasting schedules

Alternate Day Fasting

Alternate day fasting (ADF) is essentially a more advanced method of intermittent fasting. It's when you fast for an entire 24 hour period at a time. This can be once a week, sometimes twice a week, or as often as you deem fit. A common alternate day fasting schedule is 5:2. This is when you eat 5 days a week and fast for 2. You can fast for two 48 hour periods back to back, two days. Or alternate the days and split them. For example, to split the 2 fasting days. on a Monday through Sunday schedule, fast Tuesday and Friday to give yourself at least 2 full days of eating in between each fasting day. To follow the 5:2 schedule with both fasting days back to back (more efficient for Autophagy since it is reached at the 48 hr mark), eat as usual Monday, Tuesday, Wednesday, fast Thursday and Friday, eat as usual Saturday and Sunday. The 2 fasting days can be any 2 days of the week/weekend that work best for you and your schedule.

Some believe alternate fasting can be where you "fast" every other day but on the fasting day, you're allowed up to 500 calories. So you're eating but restricting calories far below your daily caloric requirement. I do not practice this and do not believe it is beneficial after researching it. Your body is receiving calories at this point, our cells aren't starved and looking for other sources of fuel and many of the fasting benefits (other than weight loss) are not achieved.

Again, you have to do what works from you, your lifestyle and your schedule. If you opt for alternate day fasting, your fasting schedule can differ every week as well. Some weeks you might want to fast on the weekends if you do not have plans and will not be tempted by food. And other weeks a weekday may be more doable for those that are not able to eat much during the work day or do not feel as hungry when busy at work. See the graph on the next page for a visual example of ADF.

ALTERNATE-DAY FASTING

DAY 1	DAY 2	DAY 3	DAY 4	DAY 5	DAY 6	DAY 7
Eats normally	24-hour fast OR Eat only a few hundred calories	Eats normally	24-hour fast OR Eat only a few hundred calories	Eats normally	24-hour fast OR Eat only a few hundred calories	Eats normally

Extended (Long Term) Fasting

Extended fasts are fasting periods that go beyond 48 hours. They can be as short as 72 hours (3 days) while some go as long as a month or longer.

Going any longer than 72 hours requires electrolyte supplementation and experience with fasting so you can recognize signals if and/or when the fast should cease. For the sake of this book, I will discuss extended fasts up to 72 hours since those are the most common and it is rare to go beyond that for the majority of the population.

Fasting for 72 hours is common and reaps all of the benefits of fasting since you surpass every fasting window mark (12 hours, 24 hours & 48 hours discussed in the chapter _The 5 Stages of Fasting_).

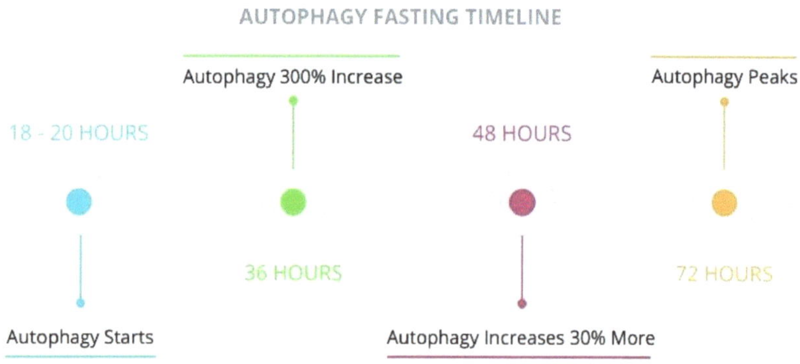

THE 5 STAGES OF FASTING

When fasting, our bodies experience growth that does not happen, or at times does not happen as efficiently and quickly, as when we regularly consume food.

When you are eating as usual, cells in your body are growing. Insulin and mTOR pathways send signals so your cells grow and reproduce. First let's understand what roles insulin and mTOR pathways play in the body.

Insulin helps the body regulate blood sugar levels in most healthy people. After you eat, carbohydrates break down into glucose, a sugar that is the body's primary source of energy. Glucose then enters the bloodstream. People with diabetes have to take insulin because their body does not adequately produce insulin this way. This is why they have to take extra caution when fasting, monitoring insulin levels very closely and stopping a fast if needed.

The mTOR pathway helps regulate metabolism. It plays important roles in the function of organs and tissue in the body including the liver, muscle and the brain. When the body is fighting a disease, such as diabetes, obesity, depression and certain cancers, the mTOR pathway is not working properly. When insulin and mTOR pathways are overactive, they can have serious implications in the body such as encouraging cancer growth.

So, how does this apply to fasting? When you are eating regularly, mTOR pathways have plenty of nutrients around, such as carbohydrates and proteins. During this time mTOR tells cells in the body not to bother with autophagy. If you recall from the chapter on Autophagy, that is when cells essentially eat & regenerate themselves. It is essentially a recycling and cleanup process that rids your body of damaged and misfolded proteins naturally.

When cells are well fed, they are not worried about being efficient and recycling its components because they are too busy growing and dividing. This is what fuels cancer growth as well.

What is important to understand is that well-fed cells have many genes, including those associated with cellular survival and proliferation, turned on. While your cells turn on cellular growth and proliferation genes when you aren't fasting, they also turn other genes off. These include genes related to fat metabolism, stress resistance and damage repair. Actually, when you fast some of your fat gets turned into ketone bodies that appear to reactivate these genes, leading to lowered inflammation and stress resistance in the brain for example.

But during starvation, things are very different. When you are fasting, your body reacts to what it sees as an environmental stress (low food availability) by changing the expression of genes that are important in protecting you from stress. We have a well-preserved starvation "program" that kicks our cell into a completely different state when food, particularly glucose or sugar, isn't around.

When you fast, and when you exercise, your body signals the cell to go into self-protective mode, activating autophagy and fat breakdown. It inhibits mTOR. This turns on genes related to antioxidant processes and damage repair throughout the body. So, a lot happens while your body isn't taking in any calories. But when exactly do these things happen? Let's look at the different stages of fasting between a 12-72 hour period

12 Hours

After 12 hours of fasting, you are at the stage called ketosis. In this state, your body starts to break down and burn fat, one of the effects of a keto diet but fasting has many more ketone benefits. Some of the fat is used by the liver to produce ketone bodies. Ketone bodies, or ketones, serve as an alternative energy source for the cells of your heart, skeletal muscle, and brain, when glucose (carbohydrates) isn't readily available. Your brain uses up some 60% of your glucose when your body is in the resting state. When you fast, ketone bodies generated by your liver partly replace glucose as fuel for your brain as well as other organs. This ketone usage versus your brain using up your glucose is one of the reasons fasting is said to promote mental clarity and positive mood.

18 Hours

By the 18 hour mark, your body is in full fat-burning mode and is generating significant ketones. If you measure your body's ketone levels using ketone strips, you can see evidence of this.

Under normal conditions, the concentration of ketones in your plasma ranges between 0.05 and

0.1 mM. When you fast or restrict the carbohydrates in your diet, this concentration can reach 5-7 mM.

As their level in your bloodstream rises, ketones can act as signaling molecules, similar to hormones, to tell your body to ramp up stress-busting pathways that reduce inflammation and repair damaged DNA

24 hours

When you reach 24 hours in a fasted state, your body is entering Autophagy. This is when your cells are recycling and regenerating themselves, breaking down misfolded proteins linked to Alzheimer's and other neurological diseases.

Autophagy is an important process for cellular and tissue rejuvenation, and aging as well. When your cells can't or don't initiate autophagy, bad things happen, including neurodegenerative diseases, which seem to come about as a result of the reduced autophagy that occurs during aging. Fasting inhibits mTOR activity, as mentioned above, which in turn activates autophagy.

This only begins to happen, however, when you substantially deplete your glucose stores and your insulin levels begin to drop. In a study of mice deprived of food, autophagy increased after 24 hours and this effect is magnified in cells of the liver and brain after 48 hours. In humans, autophagy has been detected in neutrophils starting at 24 hours of fasting. Exercise together with caloric restriction through fasting can also increase autophagy in many body tissues.

48 Hours

When you have reached 48 hours of fasting, without calories or with very few calories, carbs or protein, your body increases growth hormone production. At 48 hours, your growth hormone level is up to five times as high as when you started your fast.

The reason for this is that ketone bodies produced during fasting promote growth hormone secretion, for example in the brain. Ghrelin, the hunger hormone, also promotes growth hormone secretion. Growth hormone helps preserve lean muscle mass and reduces fat tissue accumulation, particularly as we age. It also appears to play a role in mammalian longevity and can promote wound healing and cardiovascular health.

54 hours

Once you pass the 2 day mark, at 54 hours, your insulin has dropped to its lowest level point since you started fasting and your body is becoming increasingly insulin-sensitive.

Lowering your insulin levels has a range of health benefits both short term and long term. Lowered insulin levels put a brake on the insulin and mTOR signaling pathways, activating autophagy. Lowered insulin levels can reduce inflammation, make you more insulin sensitive (and/or less insulin resistant, which is especially a good thing if you have a high risk of developing diabetes) and protect you from chronic diseases of aging including cancer.

72 hours

Three days into your fast, your body is breaking down old immune cells and generating new ones. Something crucial in today's world amidst the coronavirus.

Studies in mice have shown that prolonged fasting (greater than 48 hours) leads to stress resistance, self-renewal and regeneration of hematopoietic or blood cell stem cells. Through this same mechanism, prolonged fasting for 72 hours has been shown to preserve healthy white blood cell or lymphocyte counts in patients undergoing chemotherapy.

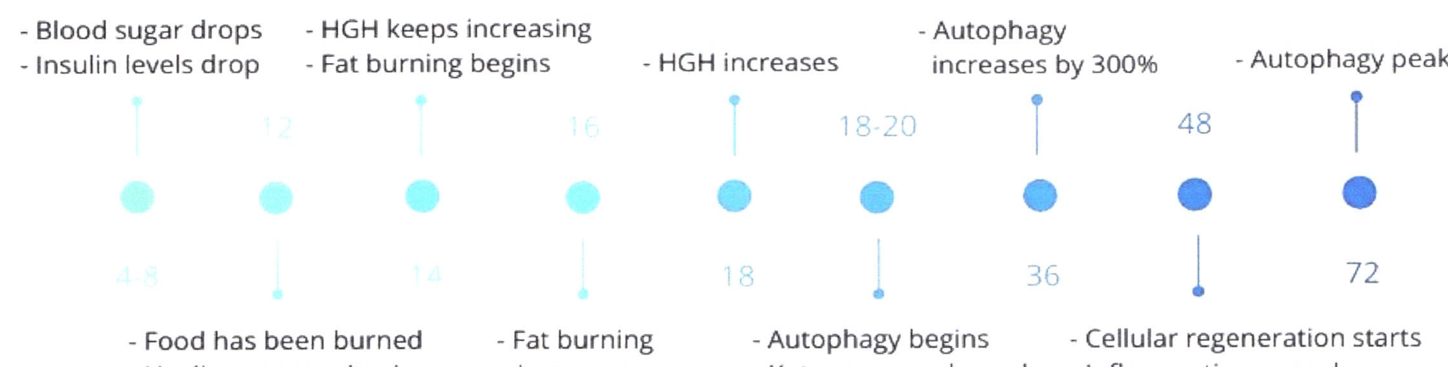
HOURLY BENEFITS OF FASTING
- Blood sugar drops
- Insulin levels drop
4-8
- Food has been burned
- Healing process begins
- HGH increases
- Glucagon is released
- Digestive system begins resting
12
- HGH keeps increasing
- Fat burning begins
14
16
- Fat burning increases
- HGH increases
18
- Autophagy begins
- Ketones are released
18-20
- Autophagy increases by 300%
36
48
- Cellular regeneration starts
- Inflammation goes down
- Autophagy peaks
72

BEFORE YOU FAST & TIPS DURING YOUR FAST

While what you eat during a fast is important, what you eat before it is important too! It's important not to binge or overly splurge for a long period of time before starting a fast. It is ok to have a "treat meal" per say, a meal of some of your favorite foods and beverages. But you should not overdo it for days before, especially eating foods high in sugar and/or refined carbohydrates.

Doing this will cause your blood sugar to spike drastically and quickly, drop quickly again, and leave you craving food, especially sugar and carbs,and possibly lead to headaches. This is much more likely to happen if you eat a high sugar diet prior to your fasting period than had you been eating a primarily clean diet. This has been my experience with fasting and I learned as I went. Doing this, and fasting in general, also helped me significantly reduce my cravings for sugar and processed carbs.

I also cannot stress enough the importance of staying hydrated, both before, during and after your fast. It helps not only keep hunger at bay, but your organs working as efficiently as possible, your digestive system moving foods that were in your body prior to the fast through and helps keep your skin supple too! A bonus most of us don't mind! This also helps avoid headaches while fasting that can be a result of dehydration.

During your fast, you will also undoubtedly experience bouts of hunger. This is, of course, part of the process of not eating. It is especially hard in the first few hours when you wake up if you are someone that is used to eating breakfast daily. It gets increasingly harder at the 16-24 mark and this is why hydration is so important. Drinking plenty of water will help keep hunger at bay. Coffee and tea help as well but be cautious not to drink it too late in the day to help you get restful sleep. And some coffee and tea are diuretics, plenty of water after consuming it is key.

Be cautious of your emotions while fasting also. Many of us are emotional eaters. We eat more so because we are stressed, anxious, depressed, etc instead of actually hungry. Fasting is a time when you should be in touch with your feelings and emotions and recognize true hunger. There will be points where you want to quit & stop the fast. Listen to your mind AND your body. If you are not feeling physically well, faint, extremely low blood sugar, etc, you may consider stopping. Headaches as part of fasting tend to be normal if you are new to fasting and proper hydration helps with this. But also stay in tune with your feelings. Stop, think, pray if this is something you do, meditate and hydrate BEFORE you give in and break your fast before you planned. As always, consult your doctor if you feel the need to prior to starting a fast.

WHAT CAN YOU EAT/DRINK DURING A FAST?

Since the point of fasting is to restrict the body's calorie intake to induce ketosis, and eventually autophagy, the list of foods, beverages and supplements you can consume for a fast is small.

IF you are fasting solely for weightloss purposes and are not interested in fasting for the health, immunity & aging benefits (although not sure why you'd do this), then you can consume more, and the list for that will be at the end of this section.

Since the purpose of this book is to share information on the many benefits of fasting outside of possible weightloss, these are the foods and beverages you can consume while fasting that will not break your fast.

- Water

- Club soda (unflavored)

- Coffee

- Green tea

- Turmeric

- Ginger

- Ceylon cinnamon

- Ginsen

- Garlic

- MCT oil (1-2 teaspoons)

- Omega-3 capsule

- Vitamins (as long as they don't have artificial sweeteners in them for flavor such as chewable a or gummies)

If you are solely fasting for weight loss, you can consume any liquid without calories such as zero calorie flavored club sodas, diet drinks & flavored coffee and teas without calories. You can also consume small amounts of fats such as coconut oil, MCT oil, heavy cream if desired.

Fasting Made Easier:

Struggling to fast consistently?
Here's a list of pantry items that can help alleviate the discomfort that often accompanies fasting.

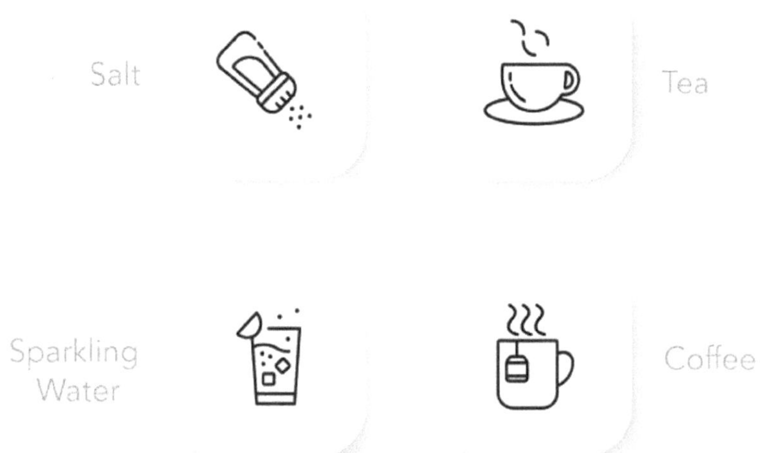

REFEEDING AFTER A FAST

One of the most important topics to understand when it comes to fasting is how to refeed once you stop your fast. It's important to break your fast with a nutritious, balanced meal that will continue to improve the function of cells and tissues that went through cleanup while you were fasting.

Having said that, it's important to break your fasts with minimal carbs and sugars to avoid problematic blood sugar spikes. Some clean, natural sources of carbs can go a long way. A balanced meal including plenty of vegetables, plant fibers and plant fats, with healthy proteins and some whole grains or legumes, is recommended. Avoid simple sugars and processed/packaged foods. Learn what works best for your body, and what you feel best eating following your fasts.

If you refeed incorrectly after a fast, your body may experience some digestive discomfort due to it slowing its production of digestive enzymes. This is often a result of eating processed foods after ending your fast, foods high in sugar and/or carbohydrates or eating large meals too quickly. The side effects often come in the form of:

* Diarrhea or loose stools

- Passing of undigested foods

- Gas pains

- Bloating

In very rare cases, nausea and vomiting. Since your body doesn't have the immediately available digestive enzymes and juices available to breakdown your food, the food can sit in your stomach much longer. It can take a few hours or more for your body to start to make what it needs to break it down. It's during this period when you may start to experience unwanted stomach pains.

Apart from shortening the duration of your fast, the best way to minimize side effects is to plan the best food to eat when you break the fast. Some people know that certain foods bother their digestive tract more than others. If you have problem foods, you should avoid them initially when you resume eating.

The recommended foods when breaking your fast are as follows:

- Plenty of water

- Plain tea or black coffee (or with stevia)

- Fresh vegetabls such as cucumber, tomato, carrots

- Leafy greens such as spinach, kale, romaine

- Poultry or fish, limit portion to the palm of your hand

- Non-starchy, above-ground vegetables that have been cooked in natural fats, like avocado or coconut oil, butter or ghee.

- Avocado

In general, the foods (and beverages) below seem to be the most problematic foods for people to consume when breaking their fast, although some tolerate them just fine.

- Nuts and nut butters

- Seeds and seed butters

- Raw cruciferous vegetables (cooked are fine)

- Eggs

- Dairy products

- Alcohol

In very rare occasions, some people have difficulty digesting certain kinds of red meat. Within six hours of ending your fast, you should be able to consume most foods without difficulty.

Avoiding alcohol, especially binge drinking, is very important when coming out of a fast of more than 36 hours. Heavy consumption of alcohol could trigger alcoholic ketoacidosis, in which ketones are very high in the blood, but unlike diabetic ketoacidosis, blood glucose is usually dangerously low.

The main symptoms are vomiting and abdominal pain. It is most common in people with alcohol addictions or strong dependence on alcohol who do not eat for a number of days and then drink heavily. However, it has been reported in individuals of all ages who have drunk heavily with little or no food intake.

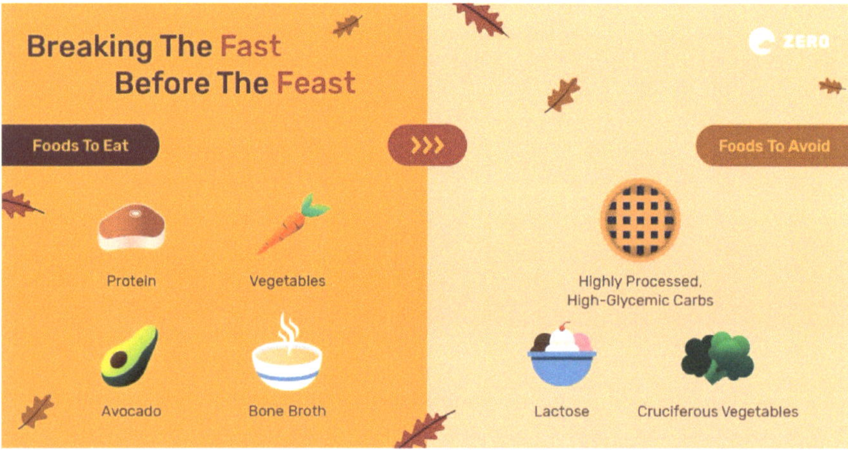

At the end of the book, you can find a 3-7 day detox meal plan that you can follow pre or post fast. It includes lean protein, healthy fats and non-processed carbohydrate choices to help your body ease out of fasting mode and continue to lose weight, minimize bloating and inflammation if that is the desired goal as well.

FASTING PRECAUTIONS

While fasting has a long list of benefits, it is important to understand that it may not be suitable for everyone. You have to do what works for your body and individual health condition. If you suffer from diabetes or low blood sugar, fasting can lead to spikes and crashes in your blood sugar levels, which could be dangerous.

Consult with your doctor and/or carefully track your blood sugar and insulin levels when fasting. Also plan to have insulin and snacks on hand and be prepared to end the fast should you feel the need to.

If you decide to try fasting, you must stay well-hydrated. It is recommended to consume at least your body weight in ounces of water each day. In addition, try to eat a diet consisting mostly of nutrient-dense foods during your eating periods to maximize health benefits.

Fasting is not recommended for children or the elderly if they have weakened immune systems unless they are closely monitored by an adult for safety reasons.

While it is ok to exercise while fasting, listen to your body. Intermittent fasting typically does not drastically affect energy levels and exercise is not usually an issue. With extended fasts for 24 hours and up, exercise can be difficult and you run the risk of nausea or fainting. Listen to your body, especially after 48-72 hrs of fasting. You may need to take the day you complete your fast off from exercise, consume nutrient dense foods, hydrate and resume physical activity the following day. See the next chapter specifically on "exercise while fasting" for more information on this topic

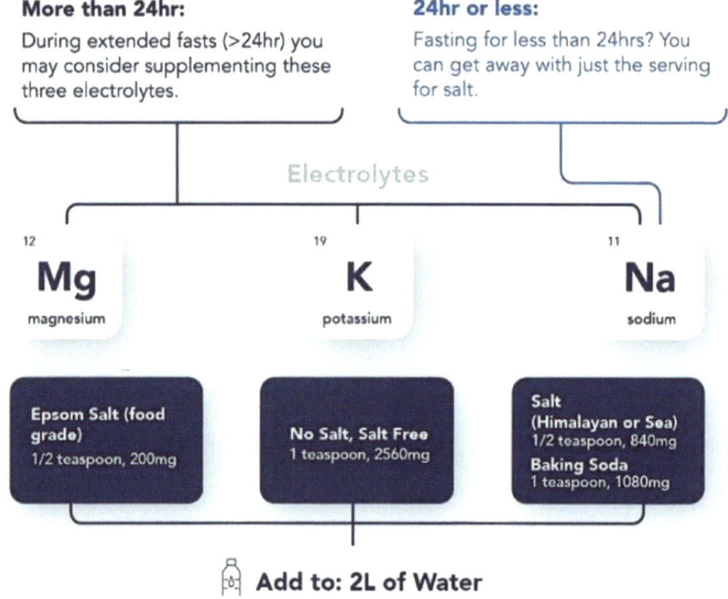

EXERCISE WHILE FASTING

Exercise is possible during a fast but it is important to use caution and listen to your body. Some people have no problem exercising while fasting, while others feel very depleted and can feel faint or lightheaded with exercise.

Like fasting, exercise creates 'healthy stress' in the body so if you are able to, you should. Research shows that exercise induces autophagy in multiple organs involved in metabolic regulation, such as muscle, the brain, liver, pancreas and adipose tissue. And moderate exercise (including a mix of cardio, resistance training and high-intensity interval training) about 30 minutes per day seems to be ideal for autophagy activation and/or increasing and improving the effects of autophagy. Alternatively, excessive or prolonged exercise could negate some of its benefits.

With that said, there are pros and cons to exercising while fasting. As mentioned above, moderate workouts no longer than 30 minutes if you do not feel depleted could actually be beneficial. But, while exercising in a fasted state, it's possible that your body will start breaking down muscle to use protein for fuel. In addition, you are more susceptible to hitting a wall, which means you'll have less energy and not be able to perform as well

Bottom Line: If you CAN and WANT to exercise, do It, it has some benefits. But make sure to do a short moderate workout and don't over exert the body when it is already being put under stress (albeit good stress) with a fast

✓ You're fasting, should you work out?

- You may burn more fat.

- If fasting long term, you could slow down your metabolism.

- You might not perform as well during workouts.

- You may lose muscle mass or only be able to maintain, not build, muscle.

FASTING APP TO TRACK YOUR PROGRESS

If you plan to start fasting, whether intermittent fasting, alternate day fasting or extended fasts, the Life app can help you keep track of your fasted vs eating times. It helps you track your fasting status and phases and also has a community where you can share your progress with others. It integrates with the Health App in your phone and also imports data from your FitBit, Garmin, Oura Ring, Biosense and other devices. You can also join fasting circles to encourage each other and hold each other accountable. The app is free and is available on the Apple App Store and the Android market

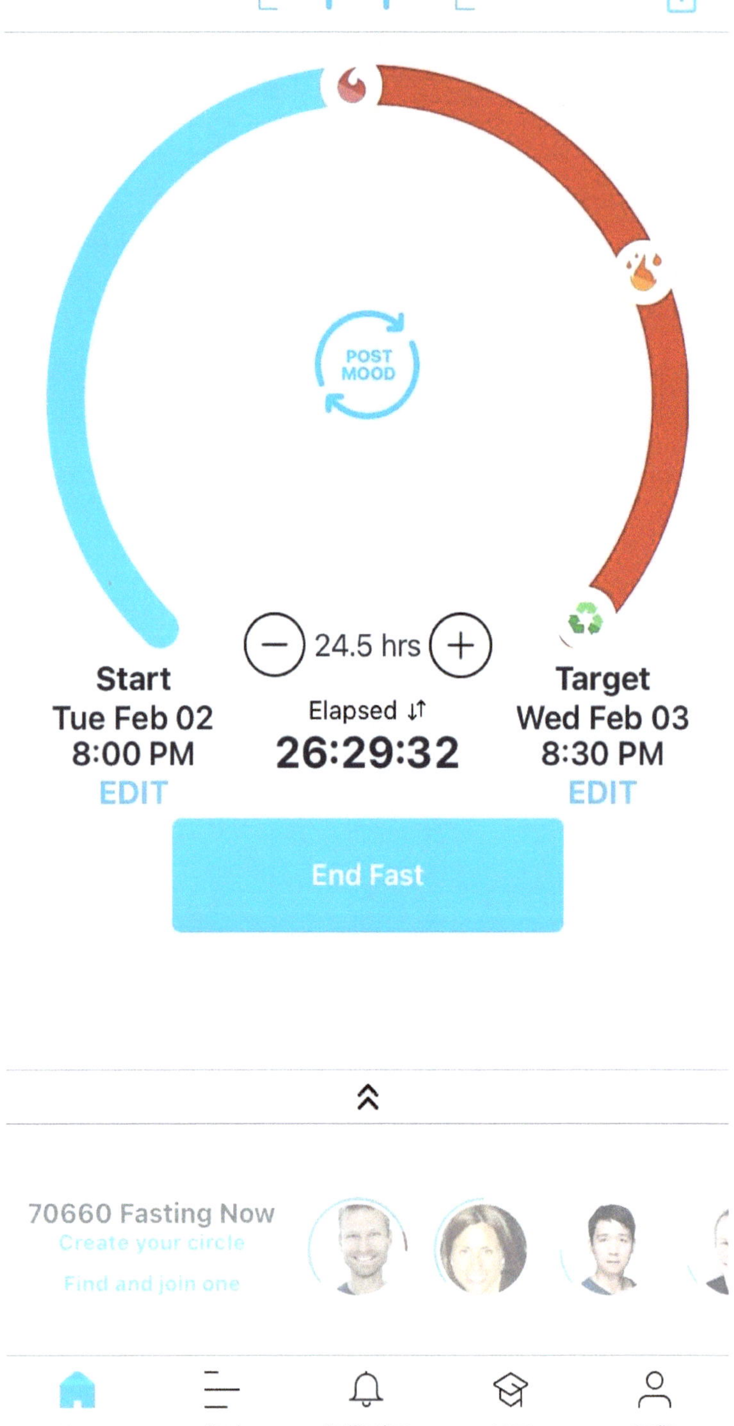

ELLIE PERICO
LIFE
POST
MOOD
24.5 hrs
Start
Tue Feb 02
8:00 PM
EDIT
Elapsed ⇅
26:29:32
Target
Wed Feb 03
8:30 PM
EDIT
End Fast
70660 Fasting Now
Create your circle
Find and join one
Home
Feed
Notifications
Learn
Profile

SAMPLE INTERMITTENT FASTING SCHEDULES

16:8 Hour Fast Normal 9-5 Schedule

Eating 12pm - 8pm

Fasting 8pm - 12 pm next day

- Wake up at 8am

    - NO EATING WINDOW 8am to 12 noon

    - Breakfast and/or Lunch at 12 noon

- Eat meals and snacks until 8pm then no eating after that

- Sleeping ideally 8 hrs then eat fast when you wake until 12pm the next day

This window can be modified if you prefer to stop eating earlier because you go to bed and/or wake up earlier. For example the eating window can be 10am to 6pm with a fasting window of 6pm to 10 am the next day. Or 9am to 5pm window with a fasting window of 5pm to 9am

16:8 Hour Fast for a Night Shift Schedule

Fasting 6am - 10pm

Eating 10pm - 6am the next day

Working approximately 10pm to 10am next day (12 hrs) Wake up at about 6pm (night shift sleep schedule)

- - NO EATING WINDOW 6pm to 10pm
  - Water, black coffee, plain green tea ok
- Late dinner/work meal at 10pm
- Eat meals and snacks until 6am during the shift then no eating after that
- Off at 10am and ideally sleep 8 hrs to 6pm and fast until 10pm again

If you have a family and prefer to eat a late dinner with them before work, you can move up your eating window to 8pm to 4am or 6pm to 2am to mimic a schedule closer to what you would do on your days off work. See a sample of this schedule below

Fasting 2am - 6pm

Eating 6pm - 2am the next day

- Eat fine before work at 6pm
- Snack & eat meals at work through 2am

- Stop eating at 2am for remainder of shift

- You can still have coffee, water, club soda and green tea Ideally you should be sleeping the next day until 12-2pm

Have a fasting window after you wake of about 4 hrs & eat dinner again to break fast at 6pm

The drawback to this type of intermittent fasting schedule for night shift worked is that you will have a long awake fasting window that includes the last 4-6 hours of your shift. It all depends on your level if hunger at work & the time you have to eat and/or drink. It also depends on how closely you want to mimic your fasting schedule on work days vs off work days. I prefer the latter (6pm to 2am) or sometimes even 5pm to 1am intermittent fasting schedule when working nights since I'm busy at work, not too hungry and really just need water and caffeine to stay awake.

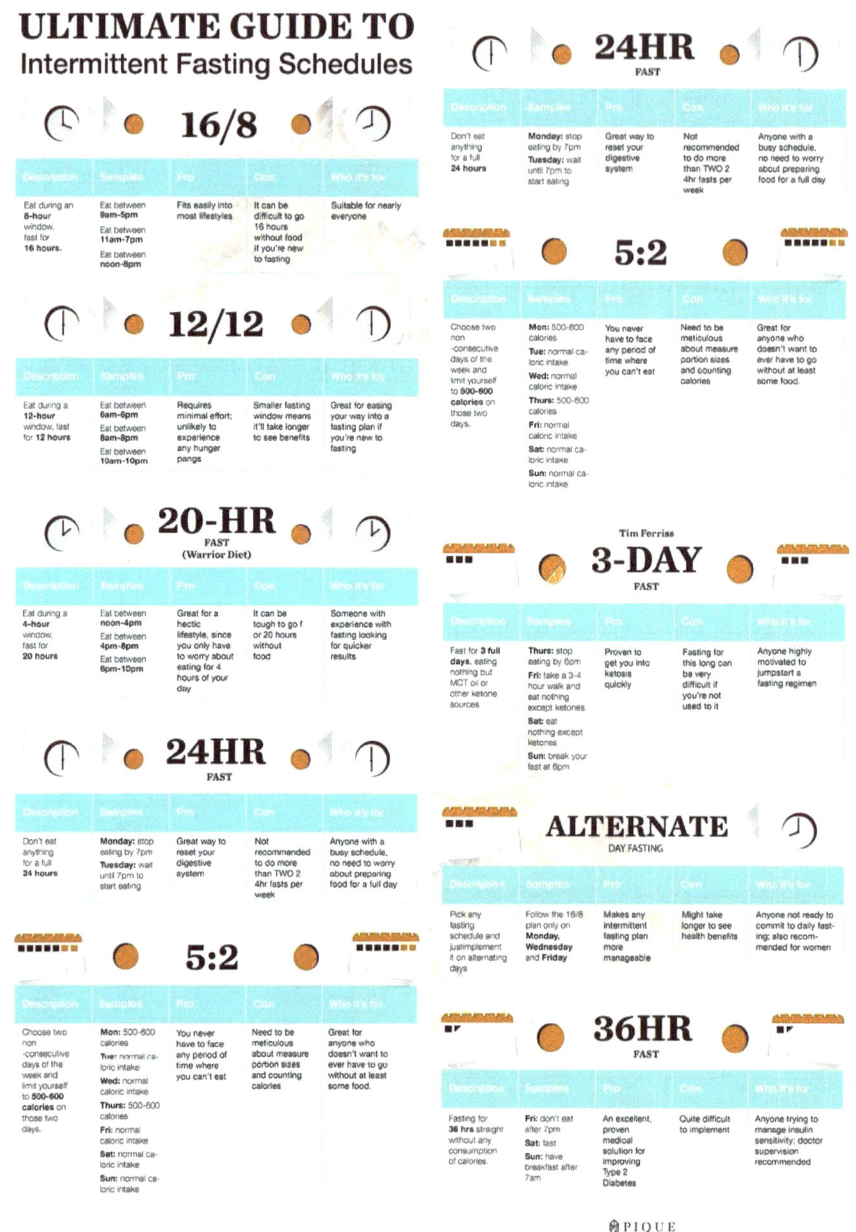

ULTIMATE GUIDE TO
Intermittent Fasting Schedules

16/8

Description	Samples	Pro	Con	Who it's for
Eat during an **8-hour** window, fast for **16 hours**.	Eat between **9am-5pm** Eat between **11am-7pm** Eat between **noon-8pm**	Fits easily into most lifestyles	It can be difficult to go 16 hours without food if you're new to fasting	Suitable for nearly everyone

12/12

Description	Samples	Pro	Con	Who it's for
Eat during a **12-hour** window, fast for **12 hours**	Eat between **6am-6pm** Eat between **8am-8pm** Eat between **10am-10pm**	Requires minimal effort; unlikely to experience any hunger pangs	Smaller fasting window means it'll take longer to see benefits	Great for easing your way into a fasting plan if you're new to fasting

20-HR
FAST
(Warrior Diet)

Description	Samples	Pro	Con	Who it's for
Eat during a **4-hour** window, fast for **20 hours**	Eat between **noon-4pm** Eat between **4pm-8pm** Eat between **6pm-10pm**	Great for a hectic lifestyle, since you only have to worry about eating for 4 hours of your day	It can be tough to go f or 20 hours without food	Someone with experience with fasting looking for quicker results

24HR
FAST

Description	Samples	Pro	Con	Who it's for
Don't eat anything for a full **24 hours**	**Monday:** stop eating by 7pm **Tuesday:** wait until 7pm to start eating	Great way to reset your digestive system	Not recommended to do more than TWO 2 4hr fasts per week	Anyone with a busy schedule, no need to worry about preparing food for a full day

5:2

Description	Samples	Pro	Con	Who it's for
Choose two non-consecutive days of the week and limit yourself to **500-600 calories** on those two days.	**Mon:** 500-600 calories **Tue:** normal caloric intake **Wed:** normal caloric intake **Thurs:** 500-600 calories **Fri:** normal caloric intake **Sat:** normal caloric intake **Sun:** normal caloric intake	You never have to face any period of time where you can't eat	Need to be meticulous about measure portion sizes and counting calories	Great for anyone who doesn't want to ever have to go without at least some food.

24HR
FAST

Description	Samples	Pro	Con	Who it's for
Don't eat anything for a full **24 hours**	**Monday:** stop eating by 7pm **Tuesday:** wait until 7pm to start eating	Great way to reset your digestive system	Not recommended to do more than TWO 2 4hr fasts per week	Anyone with a busy schedule, no need to worry about preparing food for a full day

5:2

Description	Samples	Pro	Con	Who it's for
Choose two non-consecutive days of the week and limit yourself to **500-600 calories** on those two days.	**Mon:** 500-600 calories **Tue:** normal caloric intake **Wed:** normal caloric intake **Thurs:** 500-600 calories **Fri:** normal caloric intake **Sat:** normal caloric intake **Sun:** normal caloric intake	You never have to face any period of time where you can't eat	Need to be meticulous about measure portion sizes and counting calories	Great for anyone who doesn't want to ever have to go without at least some food.

Tim Ferriss
3-DAY
FAST

Description	Samples	Pro	Con	Who it's for
Fast for **3 full days**, eating nothing but MCT oil or other ketone sources	**Thurs:** stop eating by 6pm **Fri:** take a 3-4 hour walk and eat nothing except ketones **Sat:** eat nothing except ketones **Sun:** break your fast at 6pm	Proven to get you into ketosis quickly	Fasting for this long can be very difficult if you're not used to it	Anyone highly motivated to jumpstart a fasting regimen

ALTERNATE
DAY FASTING

Description	Samples	Pro	Con	Who it's for
Pick any fasting schedule and just implement it on alternating days	Follow the 16/8 plan only on **Monday, Wednesday** and **Friday**	Makes any intermittent fasting plan more manageable	Might take longer to see health benefits	Anyone not ready to commit to daily fasting; also recommended for women

36HR
FAST

Description	Samples	Pro	Con	Who it's for
Fasting for **36 hrs** straight without any consumption of calories.	**Fri:** don't eat after 7pm **Sat:** fast **Sun:** have breakfast after 7am	An excellent, proven medical solution for improving Type 2 Diabetes	Quite difficult to implement	Anyone trying to manage insulin sensitivity; doctor supervision recommended

PIQUE

3-7. DAY PRE OR POST FAST DETOX MEAL PLAN

Before starting a fast and after completing it, it's best to eat a diet with healthy fats, lean proteins and clean carbs. This "detox" meal plan is very clean, includes 6 meals a day and is a good way to transition into and out of a fast, even if you only follow it for 1-2 days. But it can be followed for 7 or longer depending on how strict you want to be. For the first 3 days, it has to be followed exactly as it says for results (detox/weightloss). If you choose to do it for 7+ days, you can add no salt seasonings, incorporate other green leafy vegetables and have other types of fish including fatty fish such as salmon. For any other questions, feel free to email me at

ellieperico@aol.com or vía Instagram messages (@fitcopmom).

3-7 Day Detox
*Shakeoloy optional (see below)

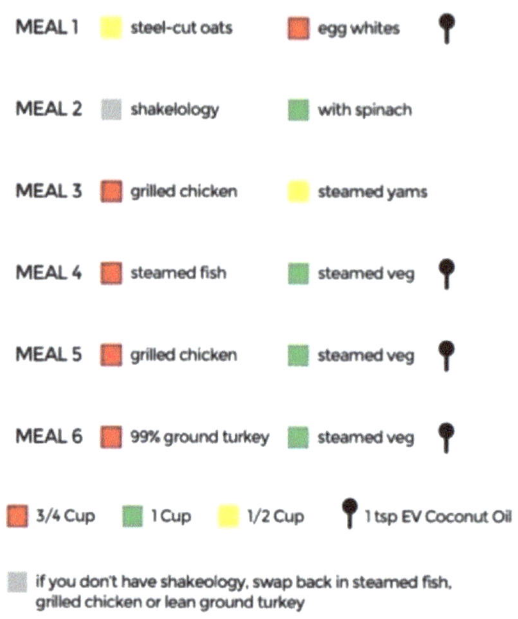

Shakeology

I use[17] shakeology as my protein shake. If you don't have it, you can replace it with steamed fish, grilled chicken or lean ground turkey as the plan states OR another comparable protein shake. Although make sure it is a clean, real food based shake such as Orgain and feel free to ask me if you are concerned it may not be comparable. I do not like the taste of Orgain and do not feel It's as beneficial so I always recommend[18] Shakeology as it has tons of nutrients, vitamins, minerals, aminos, probiotics and prebiotics as well.

---

17   https://cutt.ly/UkQnuEO

18   https://cutt.ly/QkQnvP1

If you'd like to try shakeology, there is a 7 day sampler you can try each of the flavors with and it comes with a bonus meal plan + recipes

+ workouts too! Email me (ellieperico@aol.com, send me a message on Instagram (@fitcopmom) or click on this link [19] to try it. You can get it in regular whey protein or vegan..

3-7 Day Detox Details

1. Space your meals 2 hours apart.

2. Steamed veggie options: broccoli, asparagus, green beans, zucchini, cucumbers or bell peppers

3. Seasoning options: lemon & lime juice, vinegars, herbs and spices NO SALT!

4. Oatmeal flavorings: cinnamon, nutmeg, or 1/2 tsp of stevia

5. Drink AT LEAST one gallon of water a day - spread it out as much as possible. It will help flush out the toxins.

6. Drink extra-virgin coconut oil with meals. Microwave for 10-15 seconds to get it in liquid form.

7. Coffee or tea is ok - NO creamers or sweeteners. 1/2 tsp of stevia is ok.

8. Work out as normal. But only do this meal plan for 3 days.

*Be sure to hydrate! Water consumption is crucial to your success

*If you dont want to steam your fish, you can also grill or bake it

---

19   https://cutt.ly/nkQnIdX

*If you do It for longer than 3 days and want to continue working out, do so cautiously but keep them to moderate workouts no longer than 30 minutes

3-7 Day Detox Grocery List

*this list is for 3 days. If you're doing it for 6-7 days, double the items you'll need

*egg whites are suggested if you want to substitute them for chicken, fish or turkey for any 1-2 of the meal. Fresh or frozen veggies are ok

1 small bottle of Extra Virgin Coconut Oil (12 tsp)

fresh spinach

broccoli florets*

green beans*

asparagus

zucchini

cucumbers

bell peppers

3 lbs of chicken breasts (6 breasts)

1 lbs of white fish (3-6 filets. try to stay away from tilapia)

1.5 lbs of extra lean ground turkey

1 quart of egg whites (or 1 dozen eggs separated)

Steel-cut oats

1-2 medium yams (sweet potatoes)

Thank you so much for taking the time to read the book and support my passion to teach others what I know and learn

along the way about health, nutrition and fitness. Feel free to email me any questions and/or for further help on your fitness journey!

IG | @fitcopmom FB | Ellie Perico

You Tube | @fitcopmom

FB | Health & Fitness Prívate Free Group Email | ellieperico@aol.com

9 798706 654269